MY BODY, MY RULES

I TAKE CARE OF MYSELF

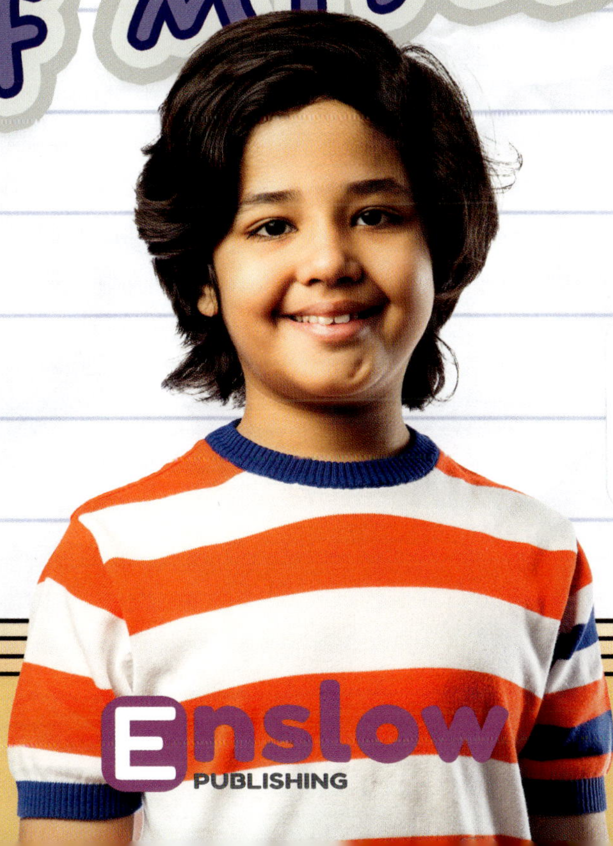

BY LAYLA OWENS

Enslow PUBLISHING

Please visit our website, www.enslow.com.
For a free color catalog of all our high-quality books, call toll free 1-800-398-2504 or fax 1-877-980-4454.

Cataloging-in-Publication Data

Names: Owens, Layla.
Title: I take care of myself / Layla Owens.
Description: Buffalo, NY : Enslow Publishing, 2026. | Series: My body, my rules | Includes glossary and index.
Identifiers: ISBN 9781978543881 (pbk.) | ISBN 9781978543898 (library bound) | ISBN 9781978543904 (ebook)
Subjects: LCSH: Self-care, Health–Juvenile literature. | Well-being–Juvenile literature. | Mind and body–Juvenile literature.
Classification: LCC RA777.O94 2026 | DDC 613–dc23

Published in 2026 by
Enslow Publishing
2544 Clinton Street
Buffalo, NY 14224

Designer: Tanya Dellaccio Keeney
Editor: Caitie McAneney

Photo credits: Series art (notebook) Design PRESENT/Shutterstock.com; series art (stickers) tmn art/Shutterstock.com; cover StockImageFactory.com/Shutterstock.com; p. 5 Q88/Shutterstock.com; p. 7 WBMUL/Shutterstock.com; p. 9 Odua Images/Shutterstock.com; p. 11 MillaF/Shutterstock.com; p. 13 Pixel-Shot/Shutterstock.com; p. 15 fizkes/Shutterstock.com; pp. 17, 19 Prostock-studio/Shutterstock.com; p. 21 Studio Romantic/Shutterstock.com.

Printed in the United States of America

CPSIA compliance information: Batch #CSENS26: For further information contact Enslow Publishing, at 1-800-398-2504.

CONTENTS

BOLDFACE WORDS APPEAR IN WORDS TO KNOW.

WHAT DO YOU NEED?

All bodies are different and special. But they need some of the same things. These include **nutrients**, water, movement, and **hygiene**. As you grow up, you can learn to take care of your body.

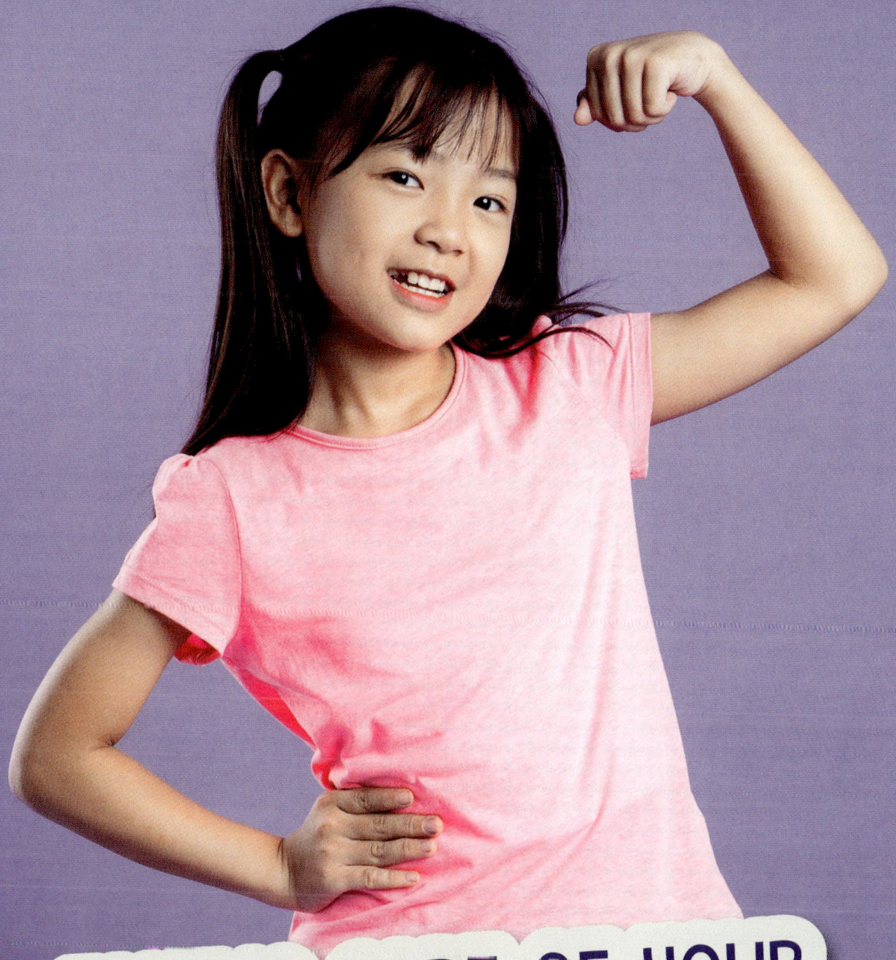

TAKING CARE OF YOUR BODY WILL MAKE YOU FEEL HEALTHY AND STRONG!

Keeping It Clean

Personal hygiene is all the things you do to keep your body clean. This can help keep you healthy. It's important to take regular baths or showers, brush your teeth, and change out of dirty clothes. Wash your hands before you eat and after using the bathroom.

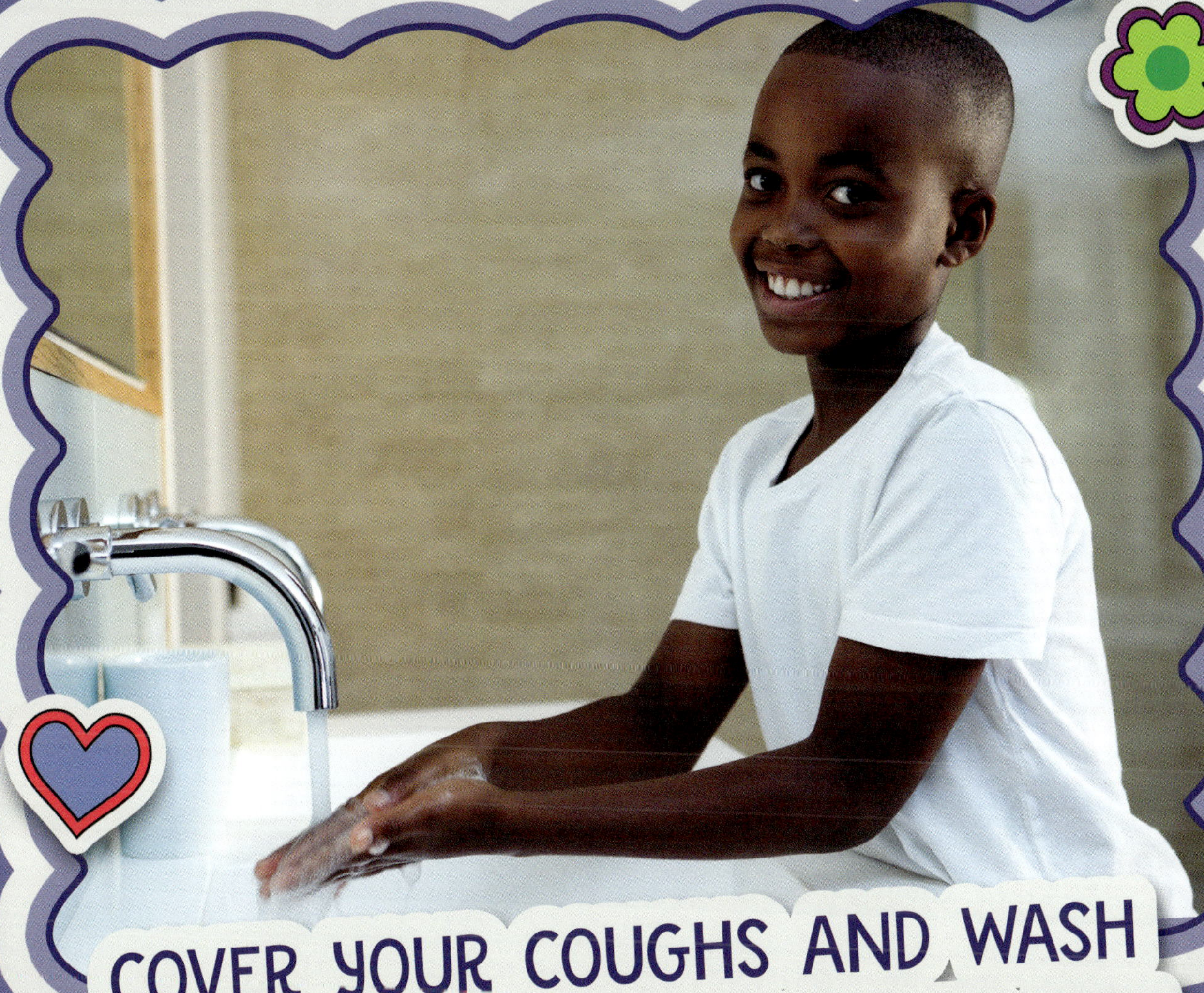

COVER YOUR COUGHS AND WASH YOUR HANDS. THIS CAN KEEP YOU AND OTHERS SAFE FROM ILLNESS!

HAZEL'S HYGIENE

Hazel has a hygiene **routine**. When she gets home from school, she washes her hands. At night, she takes a shower. She brushes her teeth and hair. She gets into clean pajamas and lays out her clothes for the next day.

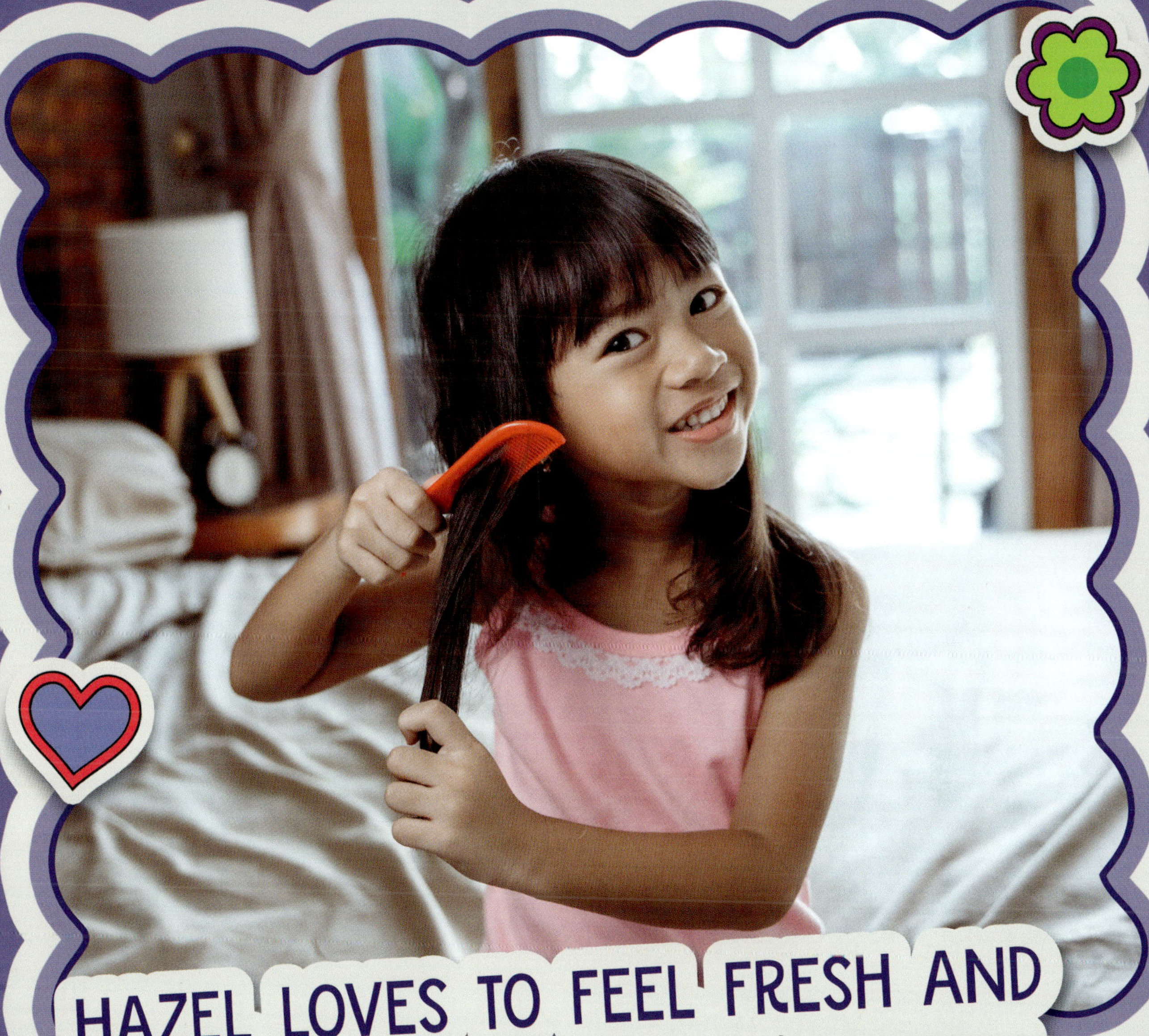

HAZEL LOVES TO FEEL FRESH AND CLEAN AFTER A DAY AT SCHOOL!

FOOD THAT FEELS GOOD

It's important to drink lots of water every day. It's also important to eat foods that have nutrients. Nutrients help your body do its work. Lots of nutrients can be found in fruits and vegetables! This kind of food makes you feel good.

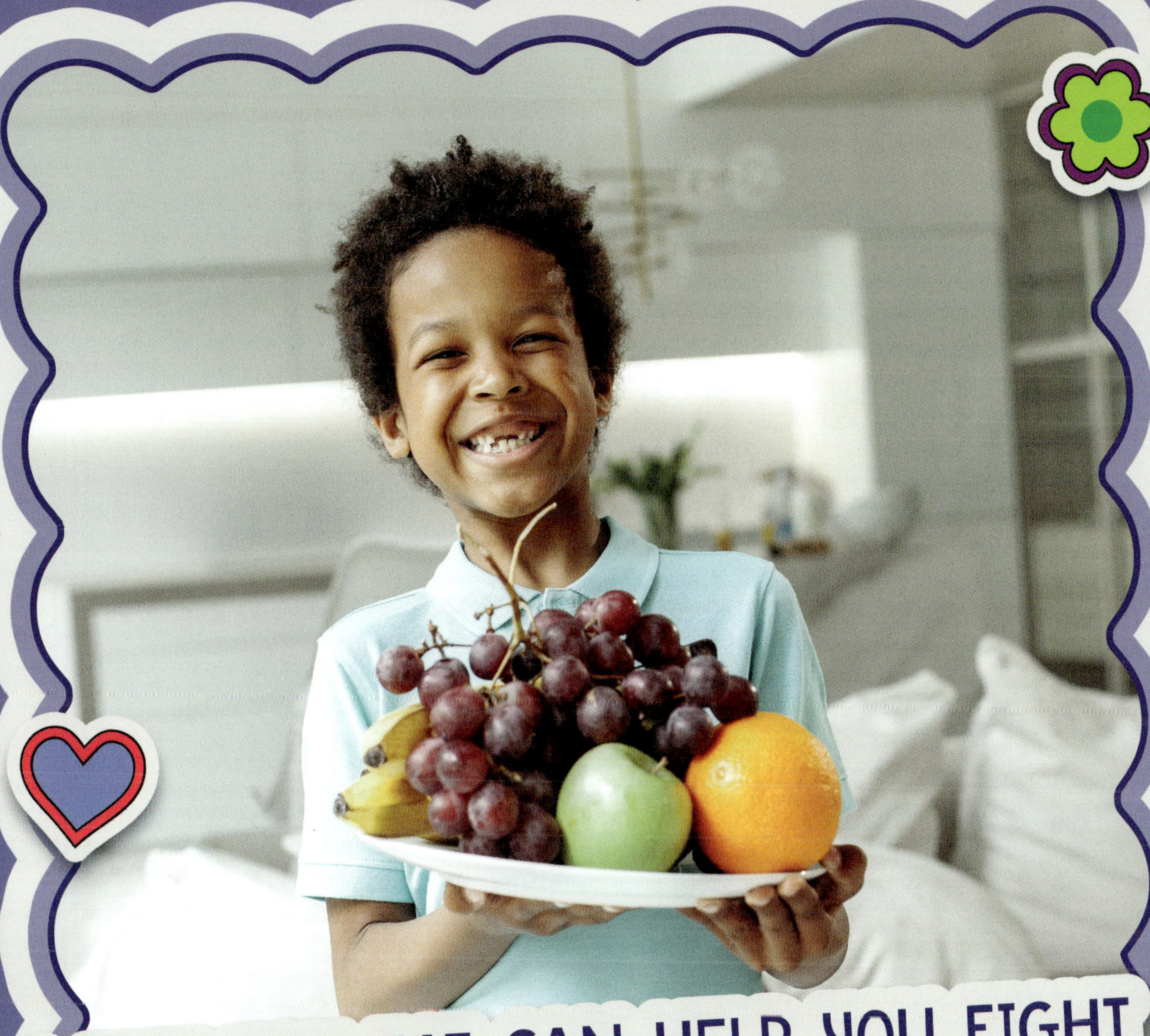

WHAT YOU EAT CAN HELP YOU FIGHT OFF ILLNESSES AND GROW STRONG.

MILES MAKES GOOD CHOICES

Miles packs his lunch. He wants to pack cookies and chips. But he knows that won't be enough to power his body. He packs apple slices, cheese, carrots, a sandwich, and a cookie. Miles also moves his body. Running makes his body feel good!

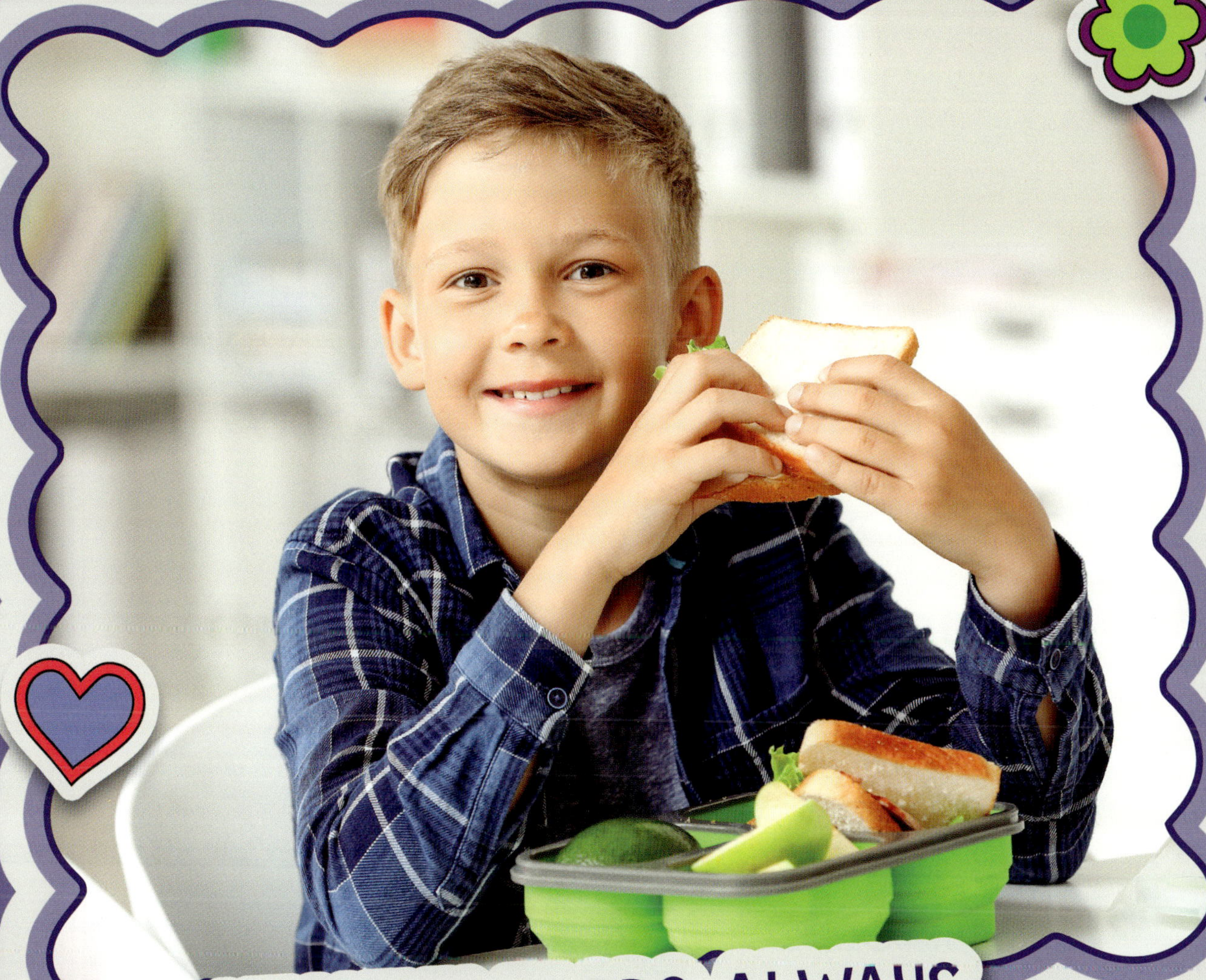

HEALTHY FOODS ALWAYS MAKE MILES FEEL GOOD.

KEEPING SAFE

You have the power to keep your body safe from harm. You can **protect** your body by wearing a helmet while biking. You can wear the right gear while playing sports. You can give clear body **boundaries** to others.

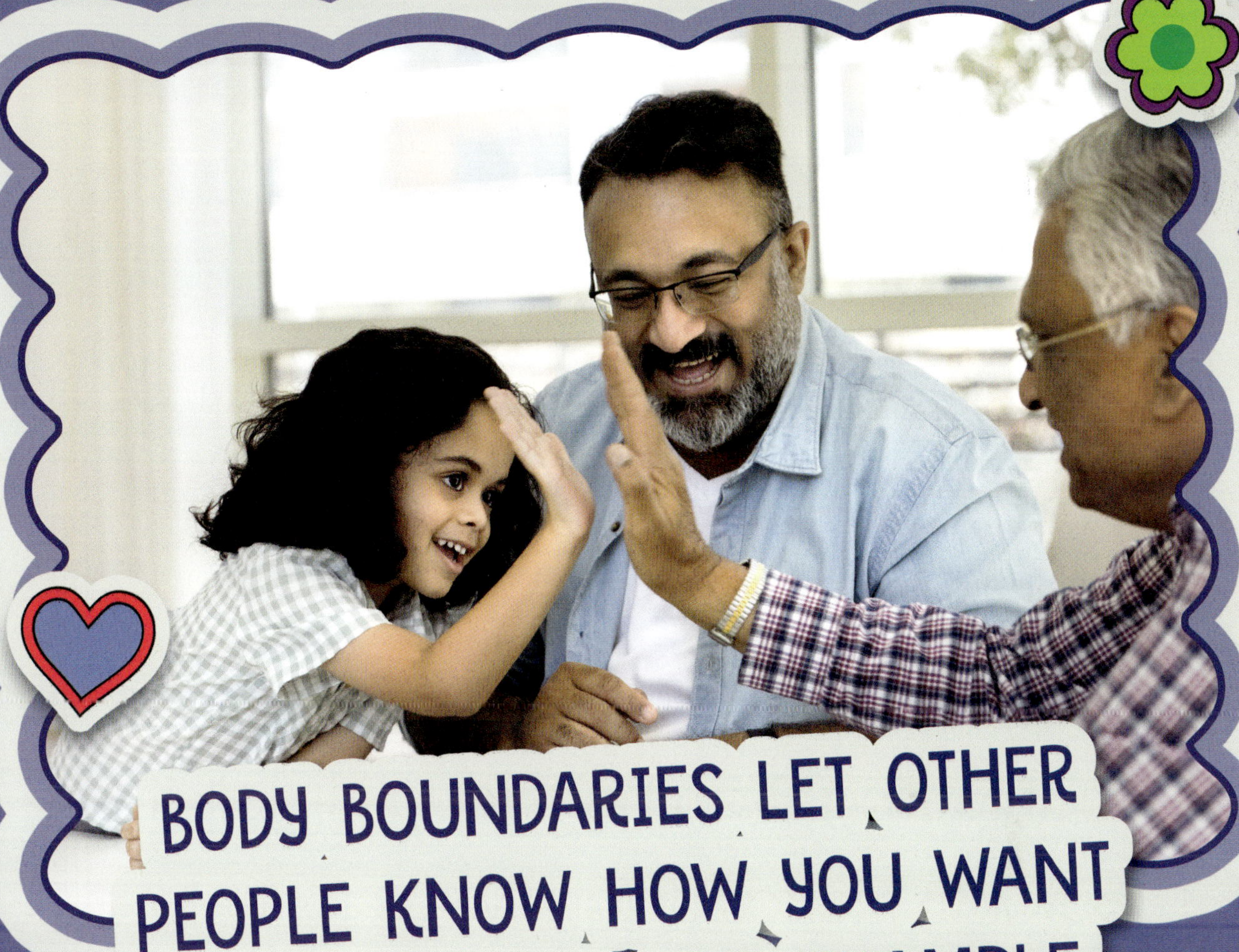

BODY BOUNDARIES LET OTHER PEOPLE KNOW HOW YOU WANT TO BE TREATED. FOR EXAMPLE, YOU MAY WANT TO GIVE A HIGH FIVE INSTEAD OF A HUG.

CARING FOR YOUR MIND

Mental health has to do with your mind, or how you think and feel. If you feel sad or mad, you can name that feeling. Breathe through it. Talk it out with friends or family. Ask for help if you need it.

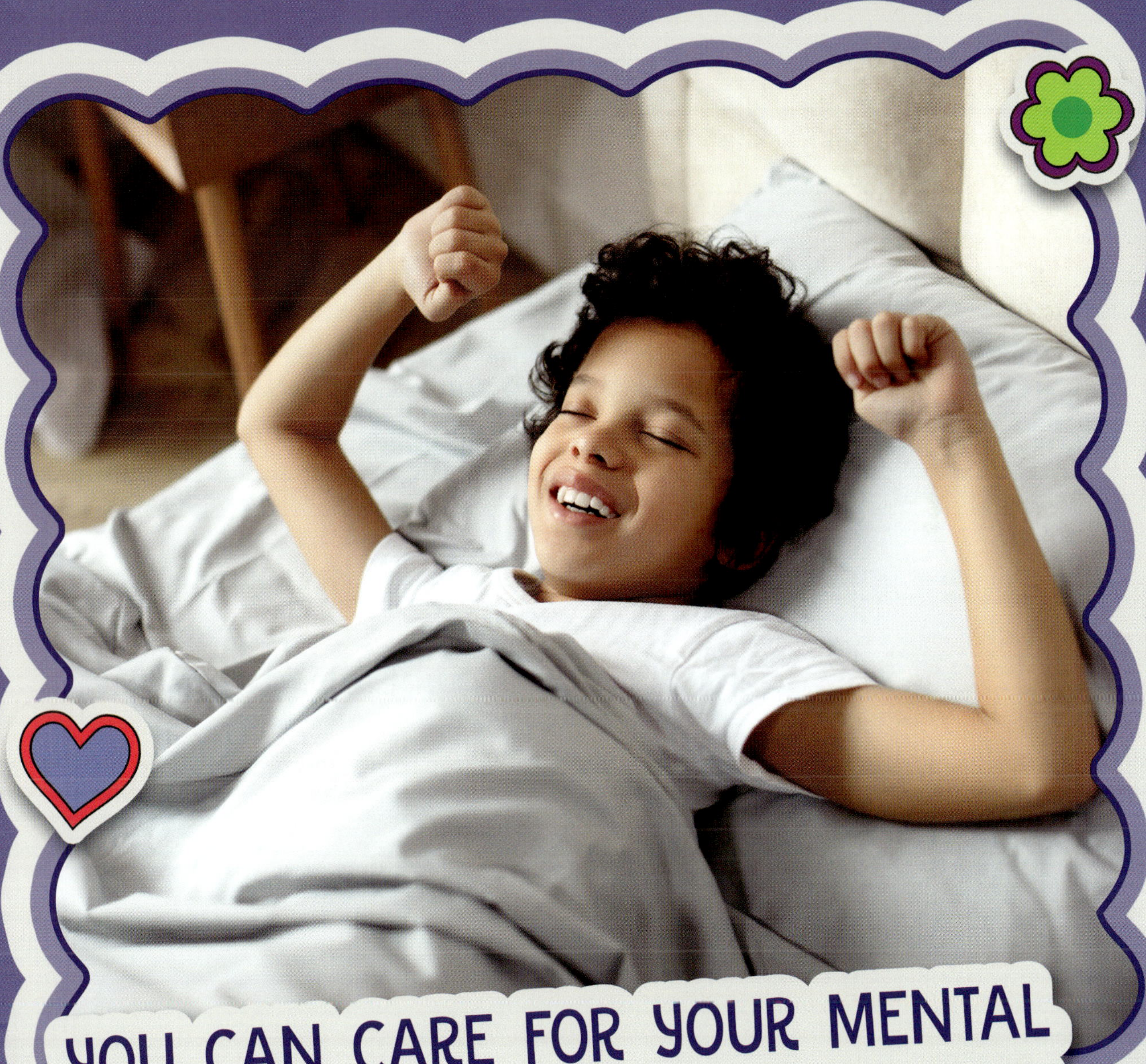

YOU CAN CARE FOR YOUR MENTAL HEALTH BY GETTING ENOUGH REST.

SUNNY'S SELF-CARE

Sunny had a hard day at school. She comes home and rests for a bit. Then she tells her sister all about her day—even the hard parts. She takes a warm bath and eats dinner. She feels better!

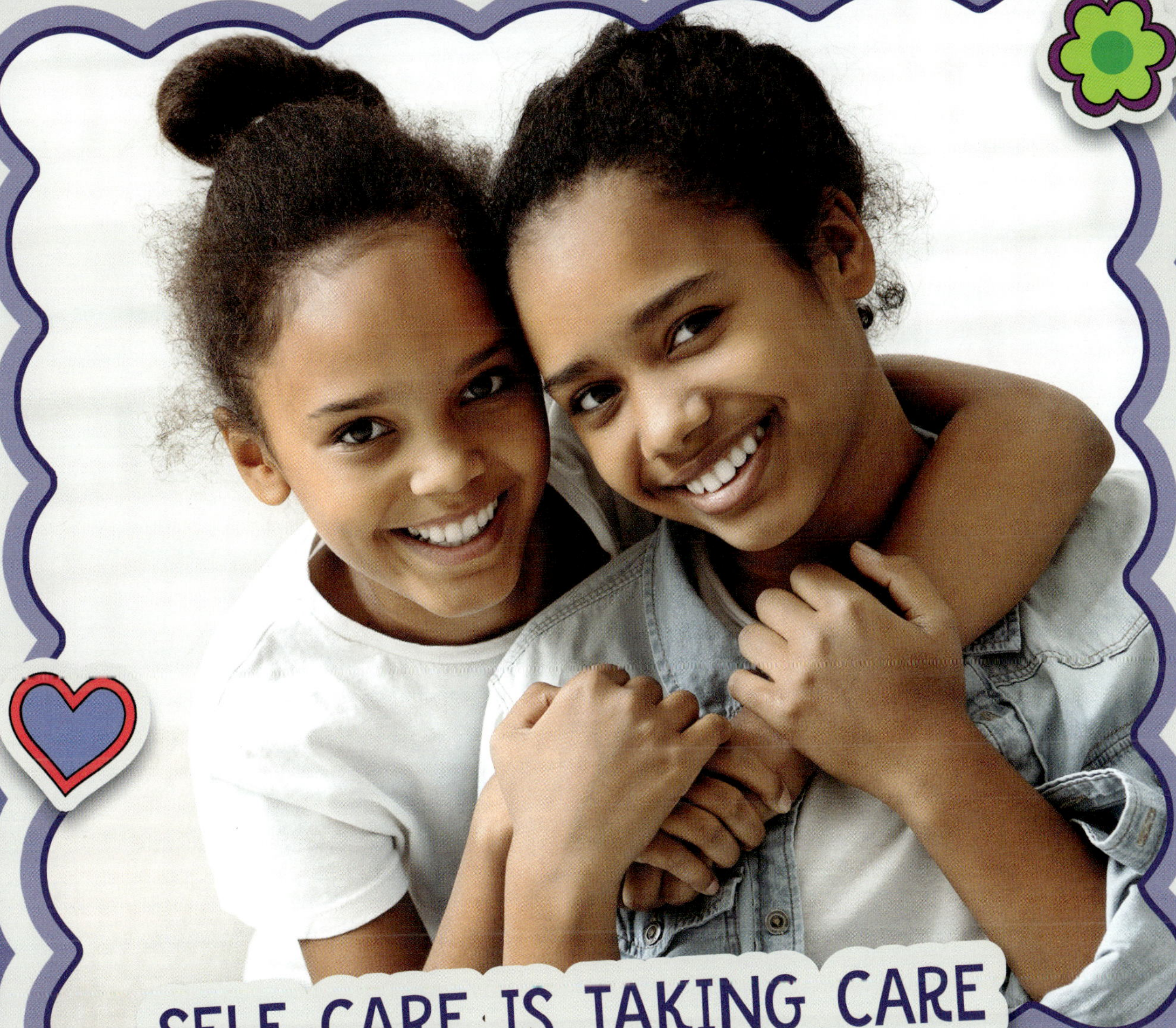

SELF-CARE IS TAKING CARE OF YOUR BODY AND MIND.

YOU ARE WORTH IT!

Your body and mind are **amazing**! It's important to care for them. Give your body what it needs. You may have hard days when you feel sick or sad. You might need a little extra care. You are worth it!

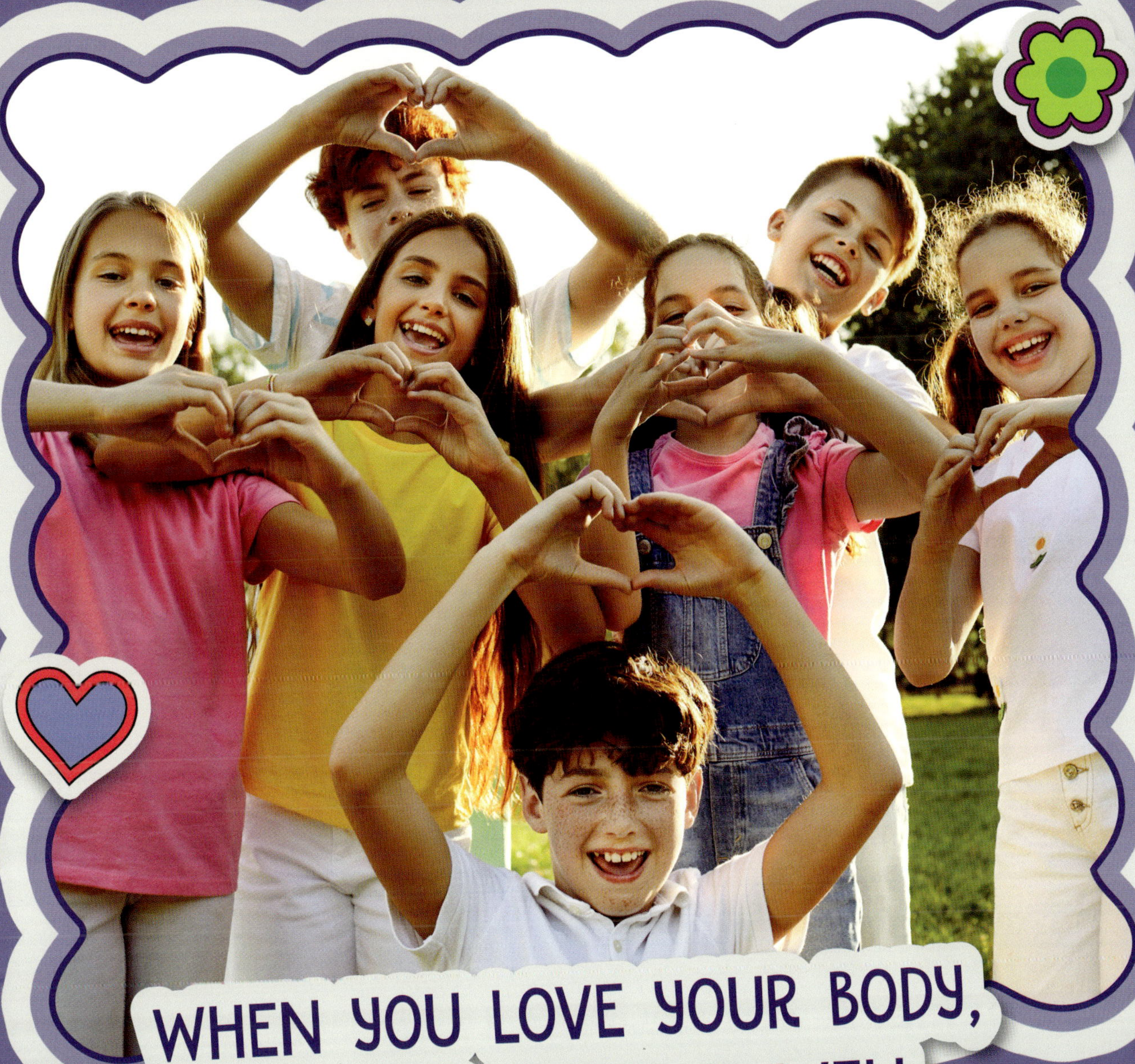

WHEN YOU LOVE YOUR BODY, YOU WILL TREAT IT WELL.

WORDS TO KNOW

amazing: Causing wonder.

boundary: A rule someone makes about how they want to be treated.

hygiene: Practices that are good for health, especially keeping clean.

nutrient: Something a living thing needs to grow and stay alive.

protect: To keep safe.

routine: A way of doing things in a certain order.

FOR MORE INFORMATION

BOOKS

Andrews, E. C. *Self-Care*. Buffalo, NY: Enslow Publishing, 2025.

Gaertner, Meg. *I Can Stop Germs.* Mendota Heights, MN: Little Blue House, 2023.

WEBSITES

MyPlate
www.myplate.gov/life-stages/kids
Learn more about how you can care for your body through healthy eating.

Why Do I Need to Wash My Hands?
kidshealth.org/en/kids/wash-hands.html
Understand how hand washing can keep your body healthy.

INDEX